**SLEEP WELL AGAIN**

# SLEEP WELL AGAIN

*How To Fall Asleep Fast, Stay Asleep Longer, And Get Better Sleep Like You Did In The Past*

## DOC ORMAN, M.D.

Copyright © 2017 by M.C. Orman, M.D., F.L.P.

All Rights Reserved. No part of this publication may be reproduced in any form or by any means, including scanning, photocopying, or otherwise without prior written permission of the copyright holder.

Calibri & Cambria fonts used with permission from Microsoft.

Published by:
TRO Productions, LLC
P.O. Box 768
Sparks, Maryland 21152

In association with TCK Publishing

www.TCKPublishing.com

Get discounts and special deals
on our best selling books at

www.tckpublishing.com/bookdeals

## Contents

Introduction .................................................................. vii

Basic Understandings About Sleep ........................... 1

Common Causes of Sleep Problems ....................... 11

How to Best Approach Solving Any Sleep
    Problem ................................................................... 17

Make Your Sleep Environment Quiet and
    Comfortable .......................................................... 35

How to Correct Bad Sleep Habits ............................ 41

Concluding Remarks ................................................ 65

Additional Resources for Sleeping Better Again ..... 67

Other Books by Doc Orman, M.D. .......................... 69

About The Author .................................................... 71

Index .......................................................................... 73

Book Discounts and Special Deals .......................... 77

## Liability Disclaimer

By reading this book, you assume all risks associated with using the advice given below, with a full understanding that you, solely, are responsible for anything that may occur as a result of putting this information into action in any way, and regardless of your interpretation of the advice.

You further agree that neither the author nor our company can be held responsible in any way for the success or failure of your sleep problem or your health or for any other aspect of your life as a result of how you choose to make use of the information presented in this book. It is your responsibility to conduct your own due diligence regarding the safe and successful application of any and all advice or suggestions offered in this book.

# INTRODUCTION

According to recent Gallup Polls, one of every three Americans suffers from occasional or frequent insomnia.

Common sleep complaints include:

- Difficulty falling asleep
- Difficulty staying asleep
- Difficulty going back to sleep after waking up at night
- Feeling drowsy or tired on awakening in the morning
- Feeling excessively tired or sleepy during the day

Similar surveys show that 20-30% of people in other countries around the world also suffer from sleep-related problems. In addition:

69% of Americans with sleep disorders never mention the problem to their physician.

26% mention it, in passing, while visiting their doctor for another problem.

Only 5% directly seek help for their sleeping problem.

Four of ten (40%) insomniacs medicate themselves to get to sleep (the most common substances used are alcohol, non-prescription sleep aids, and aspirin).

## What Is Insomnia?

Insomnia is insufficient, disturbed, non-restorative sleep.

This means not getting enough sleep to meet the needs of your body, or enough sleep to allow you to feel refreshed and energetic upon awakening and throughout the day.

## Consequences of Insomnia

The consequences of insomnia range from mild daytime drowsiness to serious injuries and even death.

Accidents can occur due to falling asleep or loss of concentration, mainly while operating an automobile or operating other dangerous machinery.

Many insomniacs report loss of ability to enjoy family and social relationships. Some avoid social contact for fear of falling asleep while visiting friends.

Far from being a benign, harmless condition, insomnia causes thousands of deaths every year. Its total cost, in

# INTRODUCTION

terms of illness, injuries, and decreased quality of life is staggering.

## How This Book Can Help

If you are one of the millions of people with chronic, recurrent, or even occasional insomnia, this book can help. In addition to providing you with a comprehensive review of basic scientific facts about insomnia, this book will also show you how to cure many of your sleep-related problems.

After completing this book, you should understand why:

- ➢ The harder you try to make yourself sleep, the less success you will have;
- ➢ The more you worry about not sleeping, the less sleep you will get;
- ➢ The longer your insomnia lasts, the more difficult it is to correct;
- ➢ Factors that caused your sleeping problem to begin may not be the same ones that are causing it to persist;
- ➢ It's easy to develop bad sleep habits that you may not be aware of;
- ➢ Sleep problems increase as you get older.

Sleeping pills are rarely the answer.

In addition, this book will also cover:

- ➢ How to diagnose the cause or causes of your insomnia;

- How to correct bad sleep habits;
- How to positively condition yourself to sleep;
- How to make your sleep environment safe, quiet, and comfortable;
- How to deal with stress more effectively;
- When and how to exercise to improve sleep;
- When to seek professional evaluation and advice.

Whatever your sleeping problem might be, most people can learn to cure or reduce their insomnia by following the principles and strategies that are discussed in this book.

## How to Get Maximum Value from This Book

This book is organized to first give you some basic information about the biology of human sleep and the typical sleep disorders that are most commonly seen.

It then reviews some of the common causes of sleep problems at a very high level. Once these important background understandings are in place, it then will give you some specific advice about how to deal with whatever sleep problem you may be having.

So the best way to get the most value from this book is to read it all the way through, from start to finish. When you come across a strategy or suggestion that might be helpful with your situation, try it out prudently, and see what results you get. Keep up with the strategies you find helpful and disregard all the rest.

# INTRODUCTION

> **KEY POINTS**
>
> Insomnia means not getting enough sleep to meet the needs of your body.
>
> One of every three Americans suffers from occasional or frequent insomnia.
>
> Four of ten insomniacs medicate themselves to get to sleep.
>
> The consequences of insomnia range from mild daytime drowsiness to serious injury and death.

# BASIC UNDERSTANDINGS ABOUT SLEEP

This chapter will introduce you to some basic information about sleep and what the term insomnia means.

## TYPES OF INSOMNIA

There are three basic types of insomnia:

1. Occasional
   (1-2 nights)
2. Short term
   (3 nights to 2-4 weeks)
3. Chronic
   (>1 month or frequent short term recurrences)

It is normal to wake up several times each night.

Although most people don't recall these brief awakening episodes, insomniacs typically have:

- ➢ Trouble either getting to sleep in the first place, or
- ➢ Trouble falling back to sleep once they have awakened.

## WHAT INSOMNIA IS NOT

The term insomnia should not be applied people who have long-standing histories of being:

- ➢ "Short sleepers"
- ➢ "Poor sleepers"
- ➢ "Light sleepers"

### *Short Sleepers*

Some people need only 3-5 hours of sleep each night to feel refreshed and energetic. These "short sleepers" do not have insomnia.

### *Poor Sleepers*

Some people never sleep well, day or night, and they've been that way most of their lives. Often, family members will have similar sleeping patterns. These "poor sleepers" may have become insomniacs early in life, but they rarely respond to usual insomnia treatments.

## *Light Sleepers*

"Light sleepers" are people who awaken easily to trivial environmental stimuli such as noise, light, or wind. In the absence of these stimuli, they have no problem sleeping and therefore do not have true insomnia.

> **NOTE:** Some people think they sleep "poorly" when in fact they sleep quite well. When their brain activity is monitored during sleep, it is often found to be completely normal despite their belief to the contrary.

Insomnia also does not apply to problems that primarily result in excessive daytime drowsiness, such as "sleep apnea" and "narcolepsy."

These disorders usually have biologic causes, and while disordered nighttime sleep patterns are sometimes involved, true insomnia is an infrequent complaint.

Significant insomnia can occur at any time. It is much more common, however, with increasing age. As people get older, they have difficulty sleeping for several reasons, which will be discussed later in this book.

Most people with insomnia have it on an occasional or intermittent basis. About 9% of the general population, however, has chronic, prolonged insomnia. Thus, at any point in time, more than 20 million Americans suffer from severe, debilitating insomnia lasting from several months to many years.

## KEY POINTS

Insomnia does not apply to "short sleepers," "poor sleepers," or "light sleepers."

Insomnia can occur at any time. However, it is much more common with increasing age.

More than 20 million Americans suffer from significant, chronic insomnia.

So far, you've learned what insomnia is and what it is not, that it's prevalent in this country and all around the world, that it has numerous possible causes, that left untreated it can have serious consequences, and that most of the time it can be successfully cured.

Now let's consider some additional background information, before going on to help you tackle your sleep-related problems.

BASIC UNDERSTANDINGS ABOUT SLEEP

## How Much Sleep Is Enough?

This varies from individual to individual. The amount of sleep that's right for you is that amount which enables you to feel wide-awake, alert, and energetic throughout the day. For most adults, this ranges between 7-9 hours, although some can feel awake and energetic on as little as 4-5 hours of sleep per night.

Researchers have discovered that normal, restful sleep in human beings consists of four patterns of brain activity called stages. Stages 1 and 2 are considered to be "light" stages of sleep, and they typically predominate in the early part of the sleep cycle. Stages 3 and 4 are deeper, more restful periods, and they tend to dominate in the latter half of sleep.

All four stages come and go many times during the night. Transient awakenings usually occur during stage 1 sleep. Most dreaming occurs during stage 4, which is also known as REM (rapid eye movement) sleep.

If the normal pattern of alternating stages is disturbed, sleep may not be fully restorative. Thus, it not only matters how many hours of sleep you get each night, but the quality of those hours and the sequence of sleep stages in your brain also play a role as well.

When our bodies are deprived of sleep at night, we generally feel tired the next day. If sleep deprivation continues, our bodies try to make up for the deficit by causing us to sleep longer at night.

> **KEY POINTS**
>
> The amount of sleep that's right for you is the amount that enables you to feel awake, alert, and energetic throughout the day.
>
> Normal sleep in human beings consists of four distinct patterns (called stages) of brain wave activity.
>
> All four stages come and go many times during the night.

## CHANGES IN SLEEP WITH AGE

It is well-known that sleep problems increase with age. As we get older, the frequency of nocturnal awakenings increases (remember, most people don't recall these brief awakenings). Changes in brain activity during sleep also occur with age. Stage 3 deep sleep progressively declines, while stage 4 (REM) sleep is relatively unaffected.

Another reason why sleep problems increase with age is that our internal biological clocks tend to change over time. These specialized brain cells located in the suprachiasmatic nucleus of the hypothalamus (a small region near the pituitary gland of the brain) control daily variations in our sleep-wake cycles.

The biological clock for most human beings cycles slightly longer than 24 hours. This is why it is easier for most people to go to bed late (since the body's sleep time is normally slightly delayed), than it is to wake up early. This also explains the problem of "jet lag," since our body's biologic rhythms become further out of synch with the social clock of the traveler's destination.

> **NOTE:** Our biologic clocks also depend upon a certain amount of daylight exposure to maintain their regulating function. This is a problem for people living above the Arctic circle, where insomnia during the dark periods of winter develops in 20-35% of the population.

As we get older, our biologic clocks gradually change. Typically, their cycle length shortens, often falling below 24 hours. This means we tend to fall asleep earlier and wake up earlier as we age. This, in turn, may lead to increased sleepiness during the day, and more daytime naps may be required.

**NOTE:** Similar, but opposite, biologic clock alterations often happen in young people around the age of adolescence. Their biologic clocks tend to lengthen beyond 25 hours, causing them to not get tired until very late at night (or early A.M.) and have trouble waking up at "normal" hours in the morning.

Thus, the changes that occur in sleep patterns with age make us more susceptible to sleep deprivation and insomnia. There is no truth to the myth that older people sleep less during the night because they "need less sleep." They sleep less because their ability to sleep may be biologically impaired, due to changes in brain functions that are beyond their direct control.

## Key Points

As we get older, the frequency of nocturnal awakenings increases.

Changes in brain activity during sleep also occur with age.

In addition, our biologic clock cycles shorten to less than 24 hours, causing us to fall asleep earlier and wake up earlier with increasing age.

There is no truth to the myth that older people sleep less during the night because they "need less sleep." They sleep less because their biologic ability to sleep becomes impaired.

# COMMON CAUSES OF SLEEP PROBLEMS

While occasional periods of poor sleep occur for just about everyone, chronic or recurrent insomnia can usually be traced to specific causes:

## 1. BIOLOGICAL CLOCK ALTERATIONS

All human beings (any many animals) have biological "clocks" deep within their brains.

These "clocks" control regular fluctuations in body functions, such as hormone secretions, temperature regulation, and sleep-wake cycles. The clock controlling sleep-wake periods typically cycles every 25 hours (interestingly not synchronized with our 24-

hour day). In some people, however, this "normal" cycle can become abnormally shortened or prolonged.

## 2. Medication Side-Effects

Prescription and OTC (over-the-counter) medications can interfere with sleep. These include decongestants, sinus remedies, diet pills, some asthma medications, and many others.

Fluid pills can cause people to wake up at night to urinate. And sleeping pills can disturb or block the normal pattern of sleep activity in the brain, thereby worsening the very problem they are designed to alleviate.

**NOTE:** Alcohol, nicotine (smoking), caffeine, and cocaine also disturb sleep patterns in the brain. These commonly ingested substances often interfere with sleep.

## 3. Withdrawal of Medications

Abruptly discontinuing certain medications, after weeks or months of use, can cause insomnia. For example, people who have been on tranquilizers or pain pills for many months can suffer from disordered sleep when they suddenly stop these medications. The withdrawal of sleeping pills causes a well-known condition called "rebound insomnia" which can last from days to weeks. And people addicted to alcohol, cigarettes, coffee, tea, or other sources of caffeine often find it difficult to sleep during acute withdrawal of these substances.

## 4. Medical or Psychological Problems

Virtually any medical or psychological problem can interfere with sleep. Painful conditions such as arthritis, gout, and acute muscle injuries are common offenders. So are illnesses that cause itching, urination, or shortness of breath at night.

Anxiety, worry, depression, and stressful life events are also extremely common causes of insomnia. In addition, medicines used to treat these conditions can also have side-effects that prevent normal sleep.

## 5. Psychological Responses to The Failure to Sleep

Another common cause of insomnia is the way people respond to their inability to sleep. After not sleeping well for several days, many people become worried, frustrated, or depressed. This causes them to place added psychological pressure on themselves to sleep. This leads to increased anxiety at bedtime, which further interferes with sleep. In no time at all, a vicious cycle of "failure--worry--more failure--more worry" develops. Once established, this failure pattern becomes self-perpetuating. It can be reversed, however, by following some of the guidelines discussed later on in this book.

## 6. BAD SLEEP HABITS

In addition to increased psychological pressure, many people fall prey to other bad habits in their efforts to restore normal sleep. Some of these bad habits include:

- Trying to "will" themselves to sleep
- Staying in bed too long while awake
- Using coffee, caffeine, other stimulants to stay awake during the day
- Oversleeping on weekends ("I'll catch up on the weekend" syndrome)

## 7. NEGATIVE ASSOCIATIONS

In addition to increased psychological pressure and bad sleeping habits, many people form negative "associations" with their bedrooms, lying in bed, lying in darkness, or other factors related to sleep. They literally learn to fear the act of sleeping. They become negatively conditioned about success in this area, and everything associated with sleep triggers unconscious expectations of failure, disappointment, shame, and humiliation.

## COMMON CAUSES OF SLEEP PROBLEMS

> **KEY POINTS**
>
> Prescription and OTC medications can interfere with sleep. These include decongestants, sinus remedies, diet pills, some asthma medications, and many others.
>
> Sleeping pills can block normal sleep activity in the brain, thereby worsening the problem they were designed to alleviate.
>
> Alcohol, nicotine, caffeine, and cocaine also disturb sleep patterns in the brain.
>
> Abruptly discontinuing certain medications can also cause insomnia.
>
> Medical and psychological problems commonly interfere with sleep.
>
> Anxiety, worry, depression, and stressful life events are also common causes of insomnia.
>
> Another common cause of insomnia is the way people respond to not sleeping well.
>
> Many people fall prey to bad sleeping habits.
>
> In addition to psychological pressures and bad sleeping habits, many people form negative associations to sleep.
>
> This book will show you how to cure many of these self-generated sleep problems.

# HOW TO BEST APPROACH SOLVING ANY SLEEP PROBLEM

The first step to approaching any sleep-related problem is to ask yourself the following five questions:

1. When, specifically, did the problem begin?
2. Is the problem mainly with getting to sleep, staying asleep, or both? (Early morning awakening, for example, is commonly—but not always—associated with stress or depression.)
3. Did the onset correspond with any unusual medical problem, psychological problem or stressful life event?
4. Did the onset correspond with any other significant change, such as starting or stopping a prescription or OTC medication?
5. Is sleep okay in other environments--hotel, hospital, or another room in your house? (If so, secondary psychological factors such as fear,

worry, performance anxiety, etc. are probably involved.)

## How to Deal with Occasional, Infrequent Insomnia

The best way to deal with one or two bad nights of sleep is to go to bed early the very next evening. Never make excuses for why you need to stay up late more than one or two nights in a row. Manage your schedule so you get your work done during the day, and don't treat your body like you can deprive it of sleep whenever you want.

Going to bed early is better for your body than taking a daytime nap. Napping during the day can make you less tired--and less able to sleep--at night. This can further interfere with resuming your normal sleep-wake cycle.

Also, don't use caffeine to keep you alert during the day or alcohol to help you get to sleep at night. Both of these substances alter the normal sleep cycles in your brain and can lead to further insomnia, which could become chronic.

It's O.K. to use prescription or OTC sleep aids to help you catch up on your sleep, as long as you use them for just one or two nights. Longer use of these substances can eventually alter the normal sleep patterns in your brain.

Also, if you need to go to sleep early, make sure your family is aware of this, so you can enlist their support in keeping your environment peaceful and quiet.

## KEY POINTS

Early morning awakening is commonly associated with stress or depression.

The best way to deal with one or two nights of poor sleep is to go to bed early the very next evening.

Going to bed early is better for your body than taking a daytime nap.

Don't use caffeine to keep you alert during the day or alcohol to help you sleep at night. Both of these substances alter the normal sleep patterns in your brain.

## How to Deal with Short-Term Insomnia (1-3 Weeks)

Longer periods of insomnia, lasting 1-3 weeks, are often precipitated by stressful life events. Repeated loss of sleep leads to poor daytime function, increased irritability, and further decreases in one's ability to cope with stress. This, in turn, leads to more worry, anger, and frustration, which additionally compromises sleep.

If you notice you are suddenly not sleeping well for several days in a row, look for recent stressful events or conflicts in your life. When you identify them, try to resolve them quickly. Don't ignore them, put off dealing with them, or simply "hope" they will go away. Address them vigorously and successfully and your insomnia will usually resolve.

Your major goal should always be to restore your previous sleep pattern just as quickly as you can. The longer insomnia lasts, the more bad habits and negative associations tend to form.

Even if you have to use a short course of sleeping pills to help you sleep, this if often preferable to allowing your body to be deprived of rest for weeks at a time. Consult with your physician before starting such a course of treatment, and make sure that you limit yourself to no more than one or two weeks of use. Again, the goal is to restore your normal sleep pattern as quickly as possible, and once this is done, your need for continued medication will generally disappear.

**NOTE:** If you do use sleeping pills for more than 7 days in a row, don't stop them all at once. Gradually decrease the dose or frequency of use, and if you have any questions about how to do this, consult with your physician.

In general, swift, aggressive, intervention can cure most types of sleeping problems that go on for several days. This can prevent long-term problems, including bad sleep habits and other negative associations, from becoming established.

Don't wait 2-3 weeks before deciding to intervene. If you haven't slept well for 3 days in a row, call your doctor and follow his or her advice. Also, be sure to use some of the other coping strategies discussed in the next section of this book.

> **KEY POINTS**
>
> Insomnia lasting 1-3 weeks is often precipitated by stressful life events.
>
> When your sleep becomes disturbed, your goal should be to restore your previous sleep pattern as quickly as you can.
>
> Swift, aggressive intervention can cure most types of sleeping problems and prevent them from becoming chronic.
>
> If you haven't slept well for 3 days in a row, call your doctor. Also, use some of the coping strategies discussed in this book.

## How to Deal with Chronic Insomnia

The best way to deal with chronic insomnia is to prevent it from becoming established in the first place. If you already have a problem that's lasted more than a month, here are some strategies most experts recommend:

### *Try to Figure Out the Cause*

Remember, insomnia is a symptom which usually has a cause. Often there are multiple causes, and the ones that initiated the problem may no longer be the ones that are keeping it from resolving. When you are trying to figure out the causes of your insomnia, consider the following categories:

### *1. Medical Illness*

Especially conditions that result in pain, shortness of breath, cough, urination, nausea, diarrhea, or other bothersome symptoms at night:

- Arthritis
- Muscle aches and pains
- Lung diseases (Asthma, etc.)
- Heart disease
- Diabetes
- Overactive thyroid gland
- Headaches
- Bowel problems (colitis, etc.)
- Heartburn or acid reflux

- Infections
- Hot flashes or menstrual pains
- Leg cramps
- Restless Leg Syndrome

**NOTE:** The Restless Leg Syndrome consists of abnormal sensations in both legs upon lying down. These sensations are usually described as "ants or insects crawling on my legs" and they are often relieved (temporarily) by moving the legs. The syndrome is also usually accompanied by periodic movements of both legs during sleep. Restless leg syndrome is a treatable problem (consult your doctor). It sometimes is associated with diabetes, kidney disease, or circulatory problems, but in the majority of cases no specific cause can be found.

## *2. Psychiatric Illness*

Any psychiatric or psychological illness can interfere with sleep. Conditions associated with increased anxiety or worry often keep people from falling asleep, whereas depressive illnesses often result in early morning awakening or trouble remaining asleep.

In addition, many prescription medications for treating psychiatric illness can also compromise sleep. Certain antidepressants, such as Prozac, Zoloft, and Paxil, can have stimulating effects. Minor tranquilizers, called benzodiazepines, may at first help anxious people sleep, but with prolonged usage they can disturb normal sleep activity in the brain. The same is true for caffeine, nicotine, and alcohol use, which frequently increase during times of psychological stress.

Also, negative associations and other bad sleep habits that become established during periods of psychological distress can remain as lingering problems after the underlying psychological crisis has resolved. For example, poor habits such as trying too hard to get back to sleep or spending too much time lying awake in bed can become established during a period of depression and remain as causes of persistent insomnia once the depression has successfully been treated (or cleared on its own).

## *3. Medications*

Prescription and OTC medicines used to treat medical or psychiatric problems can also contribute to insomnia. If you are having trouble sleeping, look very carefully at any medicines you may have been taking recently or just prior to the onset of your problem:

- Alcohol
- Caffeine (coffee, tea, colas, No Doze, etc.)
- Nicotine
- Bronchodilators (prescription drugs used for asthma and other lung diseases)
- Beta-blockers (prescription drugs used to treat high blood pressure, heart disease, migraines, palpitations, etc.)

- Prednisone or other prescription steroid medications
- Calcium channel blockers (also used to treat high blood pressure, heart disease, migraines, palpitations, etc.)
- "Non-drowsy" OTC decongestants and cold remedies (you'd be amazed how many folks take OTC meds that contain stimulants which interfere with sleep)

**NOTE:** If you are taking thyroid medication for an underactive thyroid gland, make sure to have your doctor check your thyroid hormone levels, because if they are way too high, this could be causing your sleep problem. Also, if you have no history at all of thyroid problems, but you do have an unexplained sleeping problem, be sure to ask your doctor to run some routine blood tests, including a check of your thyroid gland. Undetected thyroid problems are very common and they sometimes can be the cause of unexplained sleeping problems.

Caffeine is often used by people to maintain wakefulness throughout the day. Excessive use of caffeine on a daily basis, however, can lead to withdrawal symptoms including headache and sleeplessness at night. If caffeine is ingested too close to bedtime, its stimulating properties can also interfere with sleep. And caffeine is known to cause an increase in palpitations, stomach problems, diarrhea, and Restless Leg Syndrome in certain individuals.

Alcohol is commonly used by people to help them get to sleep. While this may appear to be a good thing to do, it eventually leads to further trouble. In addition to causing a dependency state, alcohol also disrupts the normal pattern of brain activity during sleep. While its sedative and calming effects help people get to sleep at first, it tends to produce increased nighttime awakenings and reduces the amount of Stage 3 brain activity, which is needed for proper rest.

In addition to looking at any medications or insomnia-producing substances you may be currently using, also consider any medicines you may have recently stopped! Sometimes disturbed sleep begins shortly after stopping a medication you've been taking for quite some time. For example, people who suddenly quit smoking often find that their sleep is disturbed. Withdrawing from alcohol, sleeping pills, or psychiatric medications can also produce temporary insomnia. Sometimes a more gradual tapering down of these agents will prevent this type of insomnia from occurring, so it is best to consult with your physician if you think this factor might be involved.

## 4. *Negative Conditioning and Negative Associations*

Conditioned thoughts, feelings, and behavioral responses that become associated with sleep or one's sleeping environment are common "secondary" causes of insomnia. After prolonged, unsuccessful efforts to sleep, one's bed, bedroom, turning out the lights, lying down, etc., can all become associated with failure, pain, and disappointment. As a result of these learned (but mostly unconscious) associations, increased physical and psychological arousal often occurs at bedtime. This, in turn, makes it more difficult to relax.

Insomnia-maintaining behaviors, such as staying in bed too long when you can't sleep, can also aggravate the problem. So can "performance anxiety," where the more your try to make yourself fall asleep, or the more you worry about achieving your goal, the less you are able to relax.

These "secondary" causes of insomnia are very important to recognize. One good clue is that you sleep very well in places or at times that you don't normally associate with sleep. For example, you may sleep well on vacation or at a friend's home. You may have no trouble taking unplanned naps at home, while trying to sleep at "bedtime" is often unsuccessful.

## *5. Bad Sleep Habits*

Some conditioned responses lead to bad sleep habits. These include:

- Failing to keep to a regular sleep-wake schedule
- Depriving your body of sleep by staying up to work or play on a frequent basis
- Trying to "catch up" on lost sleep during the weekend
- Watching late-night T.V.
- Excessive napping during the day

- Thinking of work-related problems while in bed
- Excessive time awareness or frequent clock-watching while in bed
- Feeling "too tired" to exercise during the day
- Exercising vigorously too close to bedtime
- Drinking tea or caffeine-containing colas close to bedtime

These behaviors commonly contribute to long-term insomnia. It's very important to recognize these causes, since in most instances they can be reduced or eliminated.

## 6. Recent Stressful Events

Another common cause of insomnia, particularly the short-term variety, is the occurrence of stressful events or crises in a person's life. These can include such events as:

- Loss of one's job
- Major changes affecting one's job
- Death/illness in relative or friend
- Being personally attacked or threatened
- Major life transitions (e.g. having a child, moving, getting married, graduating school)
- Developing a health or illness problem
- Financial crises
- Relationship conflicts
- Legal entanglements
- Committing a crime

In general, the successful resolution of these problems usually leads to restoration of normal sleep. However, if negative associations and bad sleep habits become established during periods of stress-induced insomnia, these "secondary" causes can keep one sleeping poorly.

## *7. Shift Work*

Shift work is a common cause of sleep deprivation for millions of Americans. Working the night shift on a regular basis or working different shifts on a rotating schedule produce challenges and obstacles to maintaining a normal, healthy sleep-wake pattern. This can be especially troublesome for older individuals, since the ability to tolerate shift work (from a sleep perspective) declines significantly with age.

## Key Points

Insomnia is a symptom which usually has a cause. Often, multiple causes are involved.

Restless Leg Syndrome is a treatable problem. In the majority of cases, no specific cause can be found.

Prescription medications used to treat both medical and psychiatric illness can sometimes interfere with sleep.

Negative associations and bad sleep habits that become established during times of stress can remain as problems long after the underlying crisis has been resolved.

If you are having trouble sleeping, look at any medicines you may have begun taking just prior to the onset of your problem.

Don't use caffeine close to bedtime, its stimulating properties can affect sleep.

Alcohol disrupts the normal pattern of brain activity during sleep. It produces increased nighttime awakenings and reduces the amount of Stage 3 sleep.

Sleep disturbances can also begin as a result of stopping a medication you've been taking for some time.
*cont/d...*

> Conditioned thoughts, feelings, and behavioral responses are common "secondary" causes of insomnia.
>
> Staying in bed too long when you can't sleep often aggravates the problem.
>
> It's important to recognize negative associations and bad sleep habits, since in most instances, they can be reduced or eliminated.
>
> Shift work is a common cause of insomnia for millions of Americans.
>
> If you are having trouble sleeping, make sure your sleep environment is safe, quiet, and comfortable.

# Make Your Sleep Environment Quiet and Comfortable

One thing you should always do if you are having trouble sleeping is to make sure that your sleep environment is safe, quiet, comfortable, and otherwise conducive to your personal needs for peace and relaxation.

## 1. Noise

If bothersome noises keep you awake, see what you can do to eliminate or modify their source.

If your children are the problem, get them to modify their behavior. If neighbors are the problem, see what you can do to enlist their cooperation and support. If the telephone rings late at night, try to muffle the sound, turn off the ringer, or instruct friends and relatives not to call after certain hours.

If minor noises tend to bother you, consider using a constant background noise to help you get to sleep. Some people find that an air conditioner, fan, vaporizer, dehumidifier, or other mechanical device helps to block out other distracting influences, such as noisy neighbors. Commercial devices designed to produce soothing "white noise" are also available. If these don't help, consider trying ear plugs (excellent for dealing with snoring bed partners). If all else fails, soundproofing your bedroom may be in order.

> **NOTE:** Some people need absolute quiet to get to sleep; others sleep better with mild background noise in their environment, such as T.V., radio, etc.

## 2. Darkness

If you are required to sleep during the day, too much light in your sleeping environment can be a problem. If this is true for you, consider buying thicker curtains, installing window blinds, or wearing a blindfold.

## 3. Clocks

If you are having trouble sleeping, it is best not to focus your attention on the time. This is one of the bad sleeping habits that can become a "secondary" cause of insomnia. Looking at a clock every 5-10 minutes while you are lying in bed or glancing at the clock to see what time it is each time you awaken during the night are unnecessary behaviors that should be avoided. To help you do this, consider making the following changes in your sleeping environment:

- ➢ Keep clocks and other time cues away from your bed
- ➢ No light-emitting clocks
- ➢ No ticking or chiming clocks
- ➢ Remove wrist watch at night
- ➢ Remove wall clocks or any other time device in bedroom
- ➢ If you need a clock for an alarm, get an electric one and put it out of sight (hide it under your bed, in drawer, or cover the clock face or turn the face away from you).
- ➢ Avoid focusing on time or putting yourself under time pressure of any kind

## 4. Temperature

Make sure the temperature in your bedroom is conducive to your needs. If not, consider installing an auxiliary heater, ceiling fan, air conditioner, fan, electric blanket, etc. If your temperature requirements differ from those of your sleeping partner, consider negotiating to arrive at a mutually satisfying arrangement.

## 5. General Comfort

Is your mattress comfortable? Is your pillow too soft or too hard? Would you sleep better in separate beds placed side-by-side? Would you sleep better in a queen-size or king-size bed? These and other questions of comfort should always be addressed.

## MAKE YOUR SLEEP ENVIRONMENT QUIET & COMFORTABLE

> **KEY POINTS**
>
> If minor noises tend to bother you, consider using a constant background noise to help you sleep.
>
> If you are having trouble sleeping, it is best not to focus your attention on time.

# How to Correct Bad Sleep Habits

## A. Reverse Negative Conditioning

To reverse the insomnia-producing effects of negative conditioning and poor sleep habits, consider trying one or more of the following behavior change strategies:

**NOTE:** These are often the most helpful and powerful strategies for coping with insomnia. They often require substantial patience and commitment, however, since most established habits are difficult--but not impossible--to overcome.

### *1. Create Positive Pre-Sleep Rituals*

Try reading, taking a warm bath, listening to soft music, or anything else that relaxes and pleases you on a regular basis before going to bed. Avoid any activities that might be arousing, stimulating, or worry-producing, unless they help you relax and get to sleep (e.g. sex).

## *2. Go to Bed Only When Sleepy*

Don't use your bed for any other purposes other than sleep (and sex). Do not use your bed to work, to read, to watch television, or for any other purpose. Do these things in another room, at your desk, in a chair, on the floor, etc. When you finally feel sleepy, stop these activities and get into bed. (This strategy "positively" associates your bed with feeling sleepy.)

## *3. Avoid Trying to Sleep*

By now, you should understand that the more you try to will yourself to sleep, the worse your problem will become. Remember, sleep is not a "task" to be performed. It requires a relaxed, calm, peaceful state which usually means you are not willfully trying to do anything!

If you tend to think at bedtime, don't let yourself think about work, problems, goals, projects, or other important considerations. Save these for the daytime hours, when you are more alert and can possibly do something about them.

Try to think about stupid, inconsequential, boring things instead.

**NOTE:** It is much, much easier to change the focus of your thinking than to keep yourself from thinking at all. Think about this for a minute. Now think about chickens. Now think about a quiet lake with a row boat floating peacefully on the surface. See, that wasn't hard, was it?

## 4. Establish A Regular Wake Up Time (Regardless of How Much Sleep You Get)

One of the best ways to break an insomnia problem is to establish a consistent wake up time and force yourself to stick to it seven days a week. For instance, set your alarm for 8 A.M. every day, and force yourself to get out of bed and get moving no matter how you feel at that time. Don't allow yourself to sleep later on weekends or on days when you don't have any responsibilities in the morning.

By establishing a consistent wake up time, you encourage your body and brain to adopt a consistent sleep-wake cycle. After a while, this conditioned sleep-wake pattern will take over naturally on its own.

> **NOTE:** When you first try to institute this and other strategies in this section, you may sleep worse at first. If you stick with the basic strategy, however, it will usually work out in the long run. For example, if you try to set a new wake up time but find you are waking up too early, go to bed later each night and you will soon find that the problem is corrected.

## 5. Set Aside Time to Worry (30 Minutes) Before Going to Bed

While this may sound silly, it actually works for many people! If you tend to worry excessively whenever you try to sleep, set aside a period of time (no more than 30 minutes) to get all your worrying and thinking done before bedtime. Make a list of all your immediate problem and concerns. Write down one or two actions you could take tomorrow or in the near future to help resolve them. Then go to sleep knowing that you've given serious thought to each of these problems.

If you are lying in bed and begin to think of a new problem or difficulty that you forgot to consider, get out of bed, write it down, think about it for a minute, then get back into bed and forget about it. By all means, don't allow yourself to lie in bed thinking about it. If you do continue to think about it, force yourself to get out of bed until you are finished doing so.

Some people also find that keeping a small pad and pencil by their bedside is also helpful. If they awaken during the night with a critical new thought or idea, they can quickly jot it down, thereby avoiding any worry or anxiety that they will forget it come the morning.

The bottom line is to condition yourself positively to associate your bed and bedtime with not-worrying rather than worrying. You may have to be somewhat creative to make this sort of change, but the results are very gratifying.

## 6. *Limit Time Awake in Bed*

Another very important strategy is to limit the time you spend awake in bed, particularly if you are unsuccessful at either getting to sleep or staying asleep.

If you are unable to fall asleep, don't stay in your bed for more than 10-15 minutes. Get up, get out of bed, and do something productive or enjoy-able (but not stressful or overly stimulating, such as working on your taxes, paying bills, etc.). Read, watch television, go to another room, and when you eventually feel drowsy, get back in bed and allow yourself to peacefully go to sleep. If 10-15 minutes go by again and you are still awake, get out of bed and repeat the strategy again.

If you religiously stick to this strategy, you will eventually sleep better in the long run. This is because you will be avoiding the "failure--worry--more failure--more worry" cycle that leads to negative conditioning and negative sleep associations. Even though you may lose more sleep at first and have a slight increase in daytime drowsiness (which you should expect and take precautions not to engage in dangerous activities), your sleep should eventually improve.

**NOTE:** It may take as long as 2-3 weeks before this strategy begins to pay dividends.

## *7. Try Sleeping in Different Locations*

Another useful strategy is to change your sleep environment. Since your main environment (usually your bedroom) can become negatively associated with sleep, you may find that you sleep much better in non-familiar surroundings.

Try sleeping in a guest room, on a couch in your living room, on the kitchen floor, a motel, etc. This may sound strange, but it works for many people! If you find that this helps, it should a clue that negative conditioning and negative associations are probably playing a role in your insomnia. Once you know this, you can apply some of the other strategies discussed in this section to reverse these negative patterns of thinking and behaving.

## Key Points

Try reading, taking a warm bath, listening to soft music, or anything else that relaxes you prior to going to bed.

If you are having trouble sleeping, don't use your bed to work, read, watch T.V., etc.

The more you try to will yourself to sleep, the worse your problem will become.

If you tend to think at bedtime, don't think about work, goals, projects, or other important matters.

One of the best ways to break an insomnia problem is to establish a consistent wake up time, seven days a week.

If you tend to worry whenever you try to sleep, set aside a period of time (15-30 min.) to get your worrying done prior to bedtime.

Some people find that keeping a pad and pencil by their bedside is also helpful.

If you are unable to fall asleep, don't stay in bed for more than 10-15 minutes.

Another useful strategy is to change your sleep environment.

## B. Avoid Alcohol, Caffeine, Nicotine (Especially Late in The Day)

If you are having trouble sleeping, it is best to avoid alcohol, caffeine, and nicotine altogether. For example, the caffeine you ingest from one or two cups of coffee or tea can affect your brain for 12-24 hours! Similar effects can be produced by colas, chocolate, diet pills, and other caffeine-containing substances. If you can't stay away from these completely, try not to use them after lunch.

While alcohol may relax you and help you get to sleep, it can disturb nighttime sleep activity in your brain. This can cause you to wake up more frequently during the night and fail to obtain the deep sleep that is needed to refresh you.

Smoking and other sources of nicotine (such as nicotine gum or patches) can also interfere with sleep. Nicotine is a powerful brain stimulant. When heavy smokers quit the habit, their sleep often improves in the long run.

Be careful not to abruptly withdraw any of these agents, especially if you have used them daily for months or years. Acute withdrawal reactions, and the arousal state that accompanies them, can often interfere with sleep and make your insomnia worse. For best results, consult your physician about how to gradually taper down and eventually discontinue these substances.

**NOTE:** Chronic alcoholics may have disordered sleep patterns for months or even years after cessation of drinking.

## C. Don't Nap During the Day

While napping during the day might seem tempting--and even helpful--it can also work against you. Sleeping during the day makes it harder for you to get to sleep at night. This keeps you from establishing and maintaining a regular sleep-wake cycle, which is one of your best defenses against insomnia. The failure to sleep well at night also makes you prone to develop other bad sleeping habits and negative sleep associations.

Frequent daytime napping can even reset your biological clock, thereby making it even more difficult to regain normal sleep-wake timing. For these and other reasons, it is usually better to deprive yourself of napping during the day so that you will feel more tired and sleepy at night.

**NOTE:** Some people, like the elderly, paradoxically find that napping during the day helps them sleep better at night. If this is true for you, it's fine to continue this pattern. Also, an occasional nap during the day may be fine for many individuals, just as long as it doesn't prevent the return to one's normal sleep-wake cycle.

> ## Key Points
>
> If you are having trouble sleeping, avoid alcohol, caffeine, and nicotine use.
>
> Alcohol may help you get to sleep, but it disturbs nighttime sleep activity in your brain.
>
> Napping during the day can also work against you.
>
> Frequent daytime napping can reset your biological clock, thereby making it more difficult for you to resume normal sleep.

## D. Exercise

Regular exercise can also improve your sleep. The amount and timing of exercise are both important for achieving this goal.

In general, research has shown that the best time to exercise (for the purpose of improving sleep) is six hours prior to bedtime. Thus, for most people on a normal schedule, exercising late in the afternoon or early in the evening is best.

If you exercise early in the morning or too close to bedtime, this benefit may be lost.

Exercise improves sleep by producing changes in chemical reactions throughout the body and the brain. Its effects may also be mediated by body temperature increases which occur with exercise. If you exercise too early in the day, these changes might wear off by bedtime. On the other hand, if you exercise too close to bedtime, these very same changes will be at their peak, and the resulting stimulation and body arousal may actually keep you awake!

For best results, it is good to exercise moderately for at least 20 minutes at a time, 5-6 days a week. The intensity and duration of exercise are not nearly as important as the long-term regularity of 20 minutes, 5-6 days a week, week after week, month after month, year after year.

If you are unable to exercise or are restricted from doing so for any reason, try taking a hot bath or hot tub about 2 hours (not six) prior to bedtime. The resultant increase in body temperature may give you some of the same sleep benefits that others obtain from exercise.

**NOTE:** Before you begin a new exercise program, see your physician for an examination. Also, if you experience any chest pains, shortness of breath, or other physical symptoms during exercise, consult your physician immediately.

> **KEY POINTS**
>
> Regular exercise can improve sleep. The amount and timing of exercise are both important.
>
> The best time to exercise (for improving sleep) is six hours prior to bedtime.
>
> Exercise improves sleep by producing changes in chemical reactions in your body and brain. Its effects may also be mediated by body temperature increases, which also occur with exercise.
>
> For best results, exercise moderately for at least 20 minutes, 5-6 days a week.
>
> If you are unable to exercise, try taking a hot bath or hot tub 2 hours (not six) prior to bedtime.
>
> Before you begin an exercise program, see your physician.

## E. Bedtime Snack?

Some people find that a bedtime snack helps them sleep. Others find that eating or drinking too close to bedtime keeps them awake. Since both hunger and eating too much can interfere with sleep, you will have to experiment to see what works for you. (Remember, eating close to bedtime can cause you to gain weight!)

Which types of foods are most helpful? Research dating back to 1937 shows that warm milk, with or without cookies or other food, is beneficial (although high in calories and cholesterol). Warm milk may be better than cold because of the body temperature effect noted above.

Turkey, which is high in tryptophan--an amino acid converted by the body to serotonin, a brain chemical believed to aid sleep--is also thought to be helpful. Commercial tryptophan products should be avoided, however, since previous outbreaks of health-related side effects and manufacturing impurities have occurred.

It is also best to avoid excessive liquids within 1-2 hours of sleeping. This is especially true if you have bladder problems, prostate problems, or other urinary tract conditions.

## F. OTC Sleeping Pills?

Over-the-counter sleeping aids generally contain antihistamines, which are known to induce a mild state of drowsiness. These agents are sometimes helpful for mild forms of insomnia. Care should be exercised in their use, however, since antihistamines can aggravate prostate problems and glaucoma.

## G. Shift Work

If you do shift work, you must pay more attention to your sleep routine than other people. Especially important is the need to protect your sleep environment and designated sleep time. Since most other people will be up and around during the time you need to sleep, you must keep them from interrupting you.

Napping may be useful to catch up on lost sleep, but it is best to establish a daily sleep routine and do what is necessary to maintain it religiously.

You should also avoid using caffeine or other "stimulants" while on night duty, since these can interfere with your sleep the next day. Occasional use of sleeping pills might be needed, but you should avoid becoming dependent on frequent or daily use of these agents.

## H. Learn to Deal with Stress

One of the best things you can do to prevent or eliminate insomnia is to learn how to deal with stress more effectively.

Most people experience periods of anxiety, tension, worry, or irritability from time to time. These negative emotions can build up during the day and affect your ability to rest at night. In addition, unresolved conflicts and unexpressed emotions, which many people try to suppress or ignore, can come out at night in the form of troublesome dreams or the inability to relax when going to sleep.

Medications such as tranquilizers, anti-anxiety agents, and antidepressants, which many people use when under stress, can also disturb sleep. So can the increased use of cigarettes, caffeine, and alcohol which often accompany periods of emotional and psychological upheaval.

One way to mitigate stress is to use relaxation techniques. These include meditation, biofeedback, yoga, self-hypnosis, and other relaxation skills that can be used during the day or at bedtime. These techniques don't work for everyone, but you might want to give them a try. It's best to practice with any of these techniques during daytime hours for several weeks before trying to use them at night. This will help you avoid premature failures or the disappointment that follows from excessively optimistic expectations.

Many people discover, however, that the best way to deal with stress is not by learning how to manage its symptoms, but to learn how to identify and deal with its underlying causes instead. Most stress management techniques, such as exercise, dietary changes, and relaxation procedures, only deal with symptoms. If you're worried about finances, for example, or if you're having stressful relationship conflicts at home or at work, these symptom-oriented coping strategies will usually be insufficient.

If you want to learn more about how to deal with the underlying causes of stress, I highly recommend my award-winning book, *The 14 Day Stress Cure*. This book contains many great insights and coping strategies for dealing with:

- Anger, frustration, worry, guilt, and other negative emotions
- Family and relationship problems
- Stress at work
- Stress-related physical problems
- Other types of stress, such as fear of public speaking, the stress of raising children, the stress of retirement, dealing with unexpected crises and change, etc.

> ## KEY POINTS
>
> OTC sleep aids often contain antihistamines. These can aggravate prostate problems and glaucoma.
>
> If you do shift work, avoid using caffeine or other stimulants while on duty.
>
> Learn how to deal with stress more effectively.
>
> One way to mitigate stress is to use relaxation techniques. These techniques don't work for everyone, however.
>
> The best way to deal with stress is not to manage its symptoms but to learn how to deal with its underlying causes.
>
> If you want to learn how to deal with the causes of your stress, read *The 14 Day Stress Cure*[1].

---

[1] http://geni.us/h6ULT

## I. When to Seek Medical Advice?

If you are having chronic or recurring sleep problems that don't clear up with the measures discussed above, you should consult your physician. Also, if you are feeling severely anxious or depressed, or if your sleep is being disturbed by pain or other physical symptoms, you should definitely notify your physician. You might need to be tested for a thyroid disorder, diabetes, or other medical problem. You might also need advice about pain medication, sleeping pills, antidepressants, muscle relaxants, or other prescription remedies.

Quinine, for example, is often helpful for relieving painful muscle cramps at night. Arthritis pains can be controlled or relieved by various anti-inflammatory substances. And if you have Restless Leg Syndrome, your doctor might choose to prescribe Klonopin (clonazepan), Sinemet (L-dopa), or other agents that frequently help this disorder.

Also, if you are thinking about using prescription sleeping pills, you should discuss this decision with your doctor. All major sleeping pills interfere with normal brain wave patterns during sleep. All can affect daytime functions, including memory, concentration, and rapid response times. In addition, the abrupt withdrawal of sleeping medication after prolonged--or several days of--use can lead to "rebound" insomnia.

While short-term use of sleeping medication is appropriate in certain instances, long-term use is rarely the answer. Most long-term insomnia can be corrected or controlled with behavioral, psychological, and other non-pharmacologic interventions.

Sleeping pills should definitely be avoided if you are pregnant, possibly pregnant, or are considering getting pregnant. They should also be avoided if you are elderly, if you work in a dangerous occupation, if you tend to drink alcohol, if you are taking other prescription medications, if you have severe kidney or liver disease, if you have any suicidal thoughts or tendencies, or if your bed partner complains that you snore excessively (this may be a sign of sleep apnea which can worsen with certain sleeping pills).

You should always use the lowest dose of medication that helps you to sleep, and discontinue usage as quickly as possible. Infrequent usage may sometimes be justified, but long-term administration should generally be avoided. (Never abruptly stop any sleeping medication you've been taking for some time without first consulting with your physician. In addition to rebound sleeplessness, you might also experience seizures, confusion, agitation, and possibly even death!)

**NOTE:** Some people with severe, persistent insomnia may need long-term treatment with sedative/hypnotic drugs. Since most of these drugs disrupt normal sleep activity in the brain, however, they should not be viewed as a good long-term solution.

> **KEY POINTS**
>
> If you have chronic or recurring sleep problems that don't clear up with the strategies discussed in this book, consult your physician.
>
> If you think you may have Restless Leg Syndrome, ask your doctor for advice.
>
> All prescription sleeping pills interfere with normal brain wave activity during sleep.
>
> The abrupt withdrawal of sleeping pills can lead to "rebound" insomnia.
>
> Most long-term insomnia can be corrected or controlled with non-pharmacologic interventions.
>
> Don't use sleeping pills if you are pregnant, elderly, or work in a dangerous occupation.
>
> Avoid sleeping pills if your partner complains that you have excessive nighttime snoring. This occasionally is a sign of sleep apnea, which can worsen with sleeping medication.
>
> If you do use sleeping pills, always use the lowest dose that helps you and discontinue use as quickly as possible.
>
> Never stop sleep medication abruptly. Consult with your physician about how to taper off gradually.

## J. Referral to a Sleep Center?

In most cases, referral to a sleep center is not necessary. It is most useful for people suffering from narcolepsy or a condition known as obstructive sleep apnea. Both of these disorders generally present with profound, uncontrollable daytime drowsiness, without obvious sleep disturbances.

While people suffering from the Restless Leg Syndrome are sometimes referred to sleep centers for testing, it is usually not necessary to do so. The diagnosis can usually be established from the typical history of abnormal sensations in the legs, and a trial of medical therapy can be initiated on this basis alone.

## K. Sleep Logs and Diaries

Sometimes, keeping track of sleep patterns and habits can be very helpful. A sleep log or diary can be kept at your bedside and information can be recorded each night and the following morning. Notations can be made about the time one gets into bed, time of awakening, number of hours slept, number of wake up periods remembered, coffee consumption, cigarette usage, etc.

After several days to weeks of using a sleep log or diary, certain patterns or relationships may come to light. For example, if you notice you sleep worse on days when you drink more coffee, try cutting back on your use of caffeine and use your sleep log to track the effect this has. You can also use a sleep log to track any other pattern you choose to modify.

## HOW TO CORRECT BAD SLEEP HABITS

Sleep logs increase your awareness of habits, patterns, and other sleep-related behaviors. They can be used by you alone, or they may be prescribed and monitored in partnership with your physician.

While most people don't accurately remember how long it took to get to sleep or how many times they awoke during the night, their estimates correlate well enough to spot important trends and tendencies.

You can design your own log if you want, or make use of the several sample logs you can find on the Internet. Just go to your favorite online search engine and enter the search term "sleep log." For most logs to be helpful, you must use them consistently for at least 1-2 weeks.

## KEY POINTS

In most cases, referral to a sleep center is not necessary.

Sometimes, keeping track of sleep patterns and habits with a sleep log or diary is very helpful.

Sleep logs increase your awareness of habits, patterns, and other sleep-related behaviors. They can be used by you alone, or in partnership with your physician.

# CONCLUDING REMARKS

My goal in writing this book was to give you a fairly detailed, but not exhaustive, overview of current knowledge about sleep and why people develop common sleep problems.

While there are certainly more complex understandings about sleep in general and also about sleep disorders, I wanted to focus your attention on specific things you can do to avoid or correct bad sleep habits and to make your sleeping environment more conducive to better, more restful sleep.

You may need to practice a bit with some of the behavior change strategies discussed in this book before you might see an improvement in your sleep.

Of course, if you continue to have sleep problems despite what you learned from this book, please be sure to consult with your physician.

# Additional Resources for Sleeping Better Again

If you'd like to keep up with the latest information and developments in sleep research, I recommend that you check out the two excellent resources below:

**National Sleep Foundation**

        www.sleepfoundation.org

**Doc Orman's Official Sleep Well Again Website**

        www.sleepwellagain.org

# OTHER BOOKS BY DOC ORMAN, M.D.

Stop Negative Thinking: How To Stop Worrying, Relieve Stress, and Become a Happy Person Again

The Irritability Cure: How To Stop Being Angry, Anxious and Frustrated All The Time

The Test Anxiety Cure: How To Overcome Exam Anxiety, Fear and Self Defeating Habits

The Art Of True Forgiveness: How To Forgive Anyone For Anything, Anytime You Want

The 14 Day Stress Cure: A New Approach For Dealing With Stress That Can Change Your Life

The Choice Of Paradox: How "Opposite Thinking" Can Improve Your Life And Reduce Your Stress

Stress Relief Wisdom: Ten Key Distinctions For A Stress-Free Life

The Ultimate Method for Dealing With Stress: How To Eliminate Anxiety, Irritability And Other Types Of Stress

# ABOUT THE AUTHOR

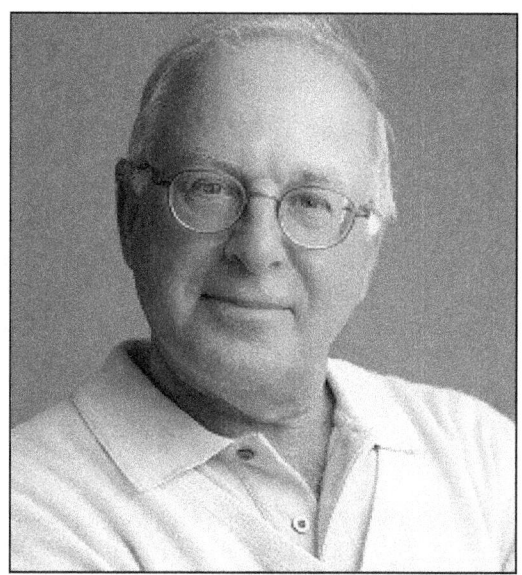

**M**ORT **(Doc) ORMAN, M.D.** is an Internal Medicine physician, author, stress coach, and founder of the Stress Mastery Academy. He has been teaching people how to eliminate stress, without managing it, for more than 30 years. He has also conducted seminars and workshops on reducing stress for doctors, nurses, veterinarians, business executives, students, the clergy, and even the F.B.I. Dr.

Orman's award-winning book, *The 14 Day Stress Cure*, is still one of the most helpful and innovative books on the subject of stress ever written. Dr. Orman and his wife, Christina, a veterinarian, live in Maryland.

You can keep in touch with Dr. Orman and find out more about his Stress Mastery Academy by visiting his website at www.DocOrman.com.

You can also follow him:

On Facebook

        www.facebook.com/beststressrelief

On Twitter

        @Doc_Orman

On LinkedIn

        www.linkedin.com/in/docorman

# INDEX

## A

accidents ..................................... viii
age, and insomnia ................ 3, 7
alcohol .......................... 26, 28, 48
anxiety ................... 13, 15, 69, 70
arthritis ....................... 13, 24, 59

## B

beta-blockers ........................... 26
biological clock ... 7, 11, 49, 50
bronchodilators ...................... 26

## C

caffeine ................. 26-27, 48, 58
calcium channel blockers .. 27
causes of insomnia ........ 24–31
clocks ........................................... 36
comfort ....................................... 37

## D

darkness .................................... 36
daylight exposure ................... 7
decongestants .......... 12, 15, 27
depression ..13, 15, 17, 20, 26
diarrhea .............................. 24, 27

diary..................*See* sleep log

## E

early morning waking......... 17
exercise................................ 51–53

## G

gout............................................. 13

## H

heart disease..................... 26, 27

## I

INSOMNIA
    causes...................... 24–31
    definition........................viii
    infrequent ...................... 18
    -maintaining behaviors . 29
    statistics .................. vii–viii
    types................................ 1

## K

Key Points......xi, 4, 6, 9, 15, 20, 23, 32, 39, 47, 50, 53, 58, 61, 64
Klonopin (clonazepan) ........ 59

## M

medical advice, when to seek............................................59

medical illness, as cause of insomnia................................ 24
medication side-effects........ 12
migraines........................... 26, 27
muscle cramps......................... 59
muscle pain............................... 13

## N

napping................ 18, 49, 50, 55
negative associations... 14, 28
nicotine................................ 26, 48
noise ........................................35–36

## O

onset, of insomnia.................. 17

## P

palpitations....................... 26, 27
prednisone............................... 27
psychiatric illness .................. 25
psychological problems....... 13

## Q

quinine ...................................... 59

## R

relaxation techniques .. 56, 58
REM (rapid eye movement) sleep............5, 7
resources ................................. 67

# INDEX

Restless Leg Syndrome....... 25, 27, 32, 59, 62

## S

shift work ............................ 31, 55
Sinemet (L-dopa) ................... 59
SLEEP
    center, referral ............... 62
    habits, poor ....... 14, 29–30
    log ............................. 62–63
    quantity ............................ 5
    stages of ........................... 5
sleeping pills, over-the-counter ........................ 54–55
sleep-wake pattern 29, 31, 43
statistics ............................ vii–viii
stress ..................... 13, 17, 55–58
stressful events ...................... 30

## T

temperature ............................. 37
*The 14 Day Stress Cure* ........ 57
thyroid medication ............... 27
thyroid problems ................... 59
tryptophan ............................... 54

## W

water pills ................................ 12
withdrawal, of medication ................. 12–13

# BOOK DISCOUNTS
## AND SPECIAL DEALS

Sign up for free to get discounts and special deals on our best selling books at

www.tckpublishing.com/bookdeals

www.ingramcontent.com/pod-product-compliance
Lightning Source LLC
Chambersburg PA
CBHW071118030426
42336CB00013BA/2137